Weight Loss for Women:

10 Proven Psychological Hacks to Lose Up to 15 Pounds in 10 Days!

Table of Content

Introduction

The human nature is a tricky sphere, which is based upon a number of various interconnected domains, we as humans sometimes get unaware about the close connections which exist between our activities and resulting aftermaths. Once these aftermaths start interrupting at their highest level we start reverse engineering to pull up the root causes. Same has happened in the case of the excessive rate of obesity. We in search of development have based our living on the fine details of the technology. For every activity there are hundreds of gadgets and appliances, hence restricting the physical activity, leading to no burn out of calories. To maximize this disaster there has been an introduction of artificial nutrition based upon hundreds of chemicals and processed food agents. The collective result is the highest rate of obesity reported, than ever in the history of mankind.

Extraneous efforts are put forward for combating the weightless issue. The market is saturated with weight loss diets and workout machines. People are also taking benefit of the services of experts but the success of all these efforts is not up to the mark. Especially the female segment suffering from obesity is highly disturbed. The reason for this turmoil is to ignore the psychological factors involved in the weight loss efforts. This book will cater weight loss from a psychological perspective so that a fuller picture can yield a clearer view.

Chapter 1 –The interconnection of Physiology and psychology- the special consideration of women psychology

The human body is a systematic orientation of various systems and biological patterns. The whole body functioning is based on an amalgamation of various bodily operations. Even the slightest change in the body's chemical and biological system can lead to serious malfunctioning. But this sensitivity is helpful in a way that it can give signals for even the slightest need for maintenance or check up.

Although hundreds of ailments and body issues are in search of human health but if you talk about the most reported issue, obesity will surely come among the toppers in the list. The modern world has transformed the living patterns and eating habits altogether. The physical activity has almost diminished from the human life, as every activity has a substitute in the form of some technological invention. The Same transformation has occurred in the eating patterns. The natural dietary elements have been replaced by hundreds of artificial flavors and 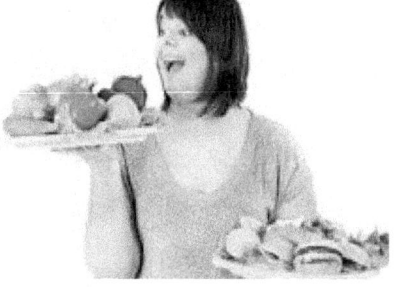 processed diet plans which have left obvious marks of obesity to people all around the planet.

Obesity has become a universal nightmare. Both men and women of all age categories are equally suffering from weight gain issues. So rather than straight away putting you into starvation techniques, it is better to understand the phenomenon with greater details. But here our focus is the female group. As among obesity victims, the percentage of women is increasing day by day.

Weight gain is both physical and psychological:

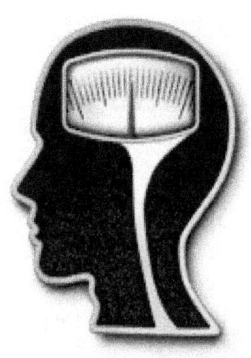

The reason for writing this book is to divert the attention of people towards the psychological domain of obesity, which has been overlooked since so long. Everyone is running behind various diet plans and exercise in order to shed pounds. But the psychological connections have been overlooked for so long. It is now time to unveil the underlying connections between the two.

Whether one is slim or fat it is considered as a physical condition of the body but the psychological impressions are also connected with it. If one is not happy from the attire and overlook of his or her body, it can have a great effect on the overall psychology of the person. It can lead to disappointment and discontentment. This virtual cycle can go a long forever, in which the person being obese becomes restless and disappointed so much so that he refrains from any kind of effort to overcome this situation. Disappointment leading to no input to the issue leads to more weight gain and it becomes a self-fulfilling prophecy.

Women are more prone to psychological traps:

Women are known to be fragile creatures that possess various distinguishing psychical and psychological features. Experts are of the view that women get more affected by obesity because they lack the control and determination which is needed during the weight loss venture.

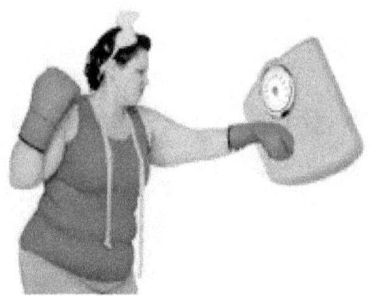

> Women are more emotional, unable to cherish emotional management for them.

> Women are more possessive about their outlook

> Women are more judgmental and compare themselves from unrealistic ideals.

> Women want appreciation and acceptance with social circles.

> The fear of losing prominence makes them feel disappointed.

Considering these important psychological aspects of women, it is important to handle the weight loss issue from a psychological aspect as well. This book is intended towards this aspect so that enough of emotional and psychological strength can be gathered thus leading towards effective weight loss. The proper diet and psychological interventions both can create miracles for any kind of weight loss issues. Diet plans followed without any include determination and psychological strength will never reveal benefit so let's consider the important psychological hacks for making up the way for weight loss.

1. Focus on the X and Y factors

2. Learn the psychological and physical domains of weight loss

3. Apply a health- belief model

4. Apply self-determination theory to your weight loss venture

5. Dig up the meaning of "Dieting"

6. Understand the barriers to "thinness"

7. Consider psychological deprivation cycle

8. Always remember about inaccurate comparisons

9. Focus on self-monitoring

10. Build up a strong support system

Chapter 2 – Apply the rules of psychology to get a "thinner" you

1. Focus on the X and Y factors

Based upon the traditional struggle which is put forward for weight loss by the majority of the victims around, you can write a simple formulaic presentation of this struggle. It will be:

$$Weight\ Shedding = Diet\ plan + workout$$

The majority of you will agree upon this. Almost all of us agree, so we try looking up the latest trends in diet plans so that we can get the best for the first part of input in the formula. Same is the case for the second part. The trendiest technology has made exercise a form of science, where every individual can get customized solution for a workout which can help him or her in gaining the optimum or ideal weight.

But this is an incomplete picture or ineffective illusion of the real picture. Weight loss is more than this, especially for women.

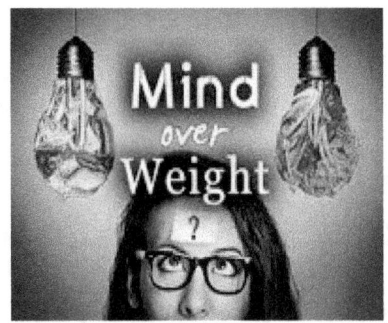

- ➤ **The corrected formula (implication of X and Y factors)**

Now if the above formula is incomplete, how can we make it correct so that the real struggle can result in obvious results. Obviously, the output side of the equation will stand still because the ultimate goal is to lose weight.

But from the input side, two significant and highly decisive factors are missing and always overlooked. Let us suppose these factors to be X and Y, such that:

Factor X = Adherence and devotion to the weight loss treatment

Factor Y = Personal change

If these factors are added to the above formula there will be no way that women will not undergo weight loss. It is the absence of these factors which lets the whole venture incomplete.

> **Adherence and devotion to the weight loss struggle**

Like any other venture or important campaign, weight loss is also a struggle. It is a fight within you, which leaves its results in the form of physical outlook and a number of pounds shown on a weight machine. But when you lack the devotion for this struggle, the diet plan and work put plans all are of no use.

First of all start with the basic questions and find the most realistic answers to these questions.

➢ Why do you want to be slim?

➢ What personal factors are involved in struggling for weight loss?

➢ What social factors are involved in struggling for weight loss?

When you will answer these questions you can easily categorize the motivational forces which can work for you. Out of these motivational forces, choose the one which can make you more devoted to the cause.

Women are known to be emotional, a bit more than men. It gives the vulnerability to get a victim of disappointment. But they need to make their selves realize that weight loss is not a game for a day or two. It is a long quest which can put up results only when followed with adherence and continuous efforts. If a woman possesses Devotion to continue fighting, she is already half the way nearer to her dream.

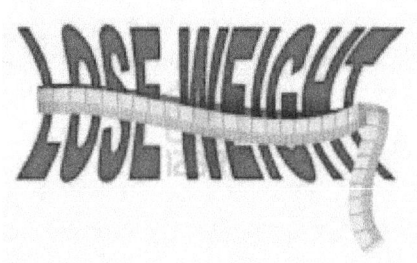

➢ **Personal change**

It is not all about starvation and keeping yourself restricted from the scrumptious and tasteful duets. Neither is it only about spending hours and hours on the treadmill. Weight loss requires a personal change. For that a woman needs to cater following important issues:

➢ What can motivate you?

➢ What is the biggest hurdle in your way of weight loss?

➢ What are top three reasons for failure?

➢ How do you learn about weight loss?

➢ Have you set specific goals for weight loss?

➢ Who are you as an individual with some specific sources of uniqueness?

➢ What your daily routine has to do with losing weight?

➢ How do you see your personality?

➢ What is the level of your defenses?

➢ What is the level of your openness?

➢ What is the level of your closed-mindedness?

➢ What is your personal history?

➢ What is the nature of your self-perception?

➢ What are the social comparisons which you make?

➢ What do you believe about your success in weight loss?

➢ What are the ways you pursue for monitoring yourself?

➢ What are the ways you pursue the feedback about weight loss results?

➢ What are the points of personal conflicts?

➢ What are your feelings regarding defeat in weight loss?

2. Learn Psychological and physical domains of weight loss

This is an extension of the corrected formula which was discussed earlier. The physical domain is related to all which you put in the form of physical struggle, like restricting yourself from eating and spending hours for physical effort. But a human body and human life cannot be fully catered if the psychological domain is left 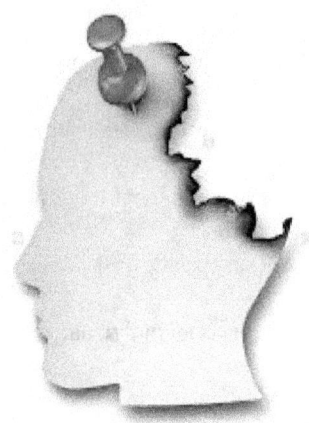 unattended. For that the psychological domain pertaining to weight loss will include following major aspects:

Self-control

Self-control is being capable of resisting the inner force which drives you against your struggle. Under self-control women will be able to cater the efforts which demand an exit out of their comfort zone so that they can put more than the standard effort. You will find clear usage of self-control when you are:

➢ Being determined to Exercise self-control

➢ Being accustomed to Saying "no"

➢ Being able to Resist temptation

➢ Having an Effortful control

➢ Resisting self-denial

- Being able to stay firm

- Putting off gratifying yourself

- Having power of mind

- Being committed your long-term goal

- Keeping the focus high

These self-control abilities will allow you to make use of physical aspects of weight loss with a greater input. In this way, you will be able to g quicker and finer results. As women are believed to be emotional and quite delicate so they give up earlier as compared to men. So this psychological hack is especially useful for women.

Self appreciation

Most of the time the biggest reason for the ineffectiveness of weight loss struggle is the inability to notice the progress. Women are usually at a higher risk of getting trapped in this phenomenon. The lack of confidence makes them unaware of their hidden talents because of which they are unable to see up the performance. Sometimes there is not a large count of pounds which needs to be given off. Only a little appreciation can make her feel better. The inability to self-appreciate is the psychological reason why women do not feel satisfied with their weight loss. If exercise and diet plan is followed with a self-appreciation about the struggle, it will lead to a motivational cycle of putting a higher level of struggles. Eventually, the results will get better with every passing day. When you will start appreciating your outlook, the devastating effects of extra pounds, if any, will also lessen. This perfect match of physical and psychological effort will leave no space for any kind of ambiguity.

3. Use health- belief model

Health belief model is a psychological model which is based on the framework of expectancy-valence. Although it is an old model, yet it has been applied recently to the concept of obesity and weight loss. Under this model, two important phenomenon reside closer to the need of attention.

➢ Locus of control

➢ Self-efficacy

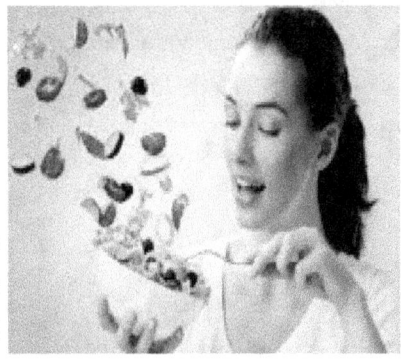

When this particular model is extended towards the weightless struggle, it narrates that one will feel motivated towards weight loss when:

(a) He has a belief that losing weight will reduce their risk of getting a life-threatening sickness

(b) He has an internal locus of control making him expect that his or her self-effort will direct specific behaviors which will result in obvious weight loss.

(c) He is confident that he is able to carry out the behaviors and activities which are mandatory for weight loss.

These points clearly predict that valuing a particular outcome, which in this case is the attainment of ideal weight through weight loss activities, and believing one's self to be able to achieve that result uphold motivation.

Here the critical point is to look up for various types of motivation

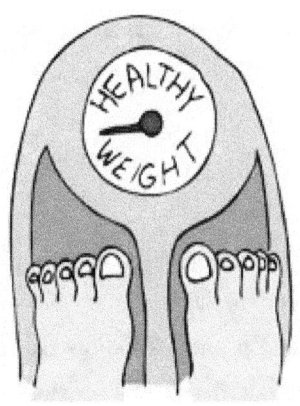

> **Autonomous motivation**

The famous self-determination theory of psychology states that autonomous behaviors are the ones for which the guideline is practiced as chosen and as appearing from one's self. Being connected to inner being of the individual autonomous motivation is related to the internal locus of control and causality also takes place from within

> **Controlled motivation**

Under the effect of controlled motivation, behaviors are said to be *controlled* behaviors for which the regulation is experienced as forced or pressured or by some external intra-psychic force or interpersonal factor. Hence, it is related to the external locus of control.

So applying these psychological principles to your weightless activity you will find new principles of successful weight loss. These principles related to the long-term maintenance of weight loss, which would *not* result from merely dieting if the reasons extended for dieting were purely controlling. So if a woman is going to gym only because his spouse wanted her to be slim and she feels guilty of not doing so, then her motivation for Weight lose activity is purely controlled. Here the external locus of control will come into play and that woman will not be able to endorse the behavior personally. The willingness to go to the gym will not be personal. Here the activity will be pursued as a burden and hence the result will also be limited.

On the flip side, if the motivation for the same activity would have come from within, then the same women would have pursued weight loss with more control and passion. This internal motivation can be developed by creating awareness about the health benefits associated with optimum weight or by having an internal desire to look young and fit. The same activity will yield fruitful results. So if you are not getting effective results, you need to look for these ways.

4. Apply self-determination theory

This is another important psychological domain which can be extended to the issue of weight loss which people are facing. This theory connotes that the regulation of a particular behavior of
a person depends on upon

➢ Individual difference

➢ Social-context variables

In this case, the focus of attention is to see the behaviors and set of activities related to weight loss, this may include following specific diets and pursuing work out session.

Within the individual difference orientation which leads to regulation of behavior, the person will have three major concepts

➢ The autonomy

➢ The control

➢ Impersonal orientation

The autonomy perspective for weight loss complies that there is always a general ability 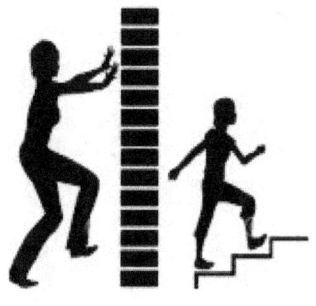 to be self-regulating in losing weight and to learn the contextual factors that endorse individual choice and personal initiative.

Autonomy orientation applied to weight loss will also create other positive behaviors like self-actualization, integration of personality and self-esteem. In this case, all those contextual factors which relate to this inner motivation will be seen as a support mechanism and person can continue with weight loss activities. Whenever this autonomous perspective will loosen the grip, the chances of getting back are greatly enhanced.

Now self-determination applies that all those women who are not finding the positive or visible result of their weight loss activity, need to internalize their effort, whenever they will pursue dieting or exercise as a pressure, they will never be able to get the maximum behavior.

You may have seen people who have maintained their weight and exercising routine for the past so many years. It is because they had developed an internal passion for doing so, in earlier years of their struggle and now the waves of motivation come from within.

Stand in front of the mirror, look up yourself and put up a dialogue with your own self. Convince and motivate yourself about pursuing weight loss venture. Extend reasons and maintain and evaluative feedback loop.

Chapter 3 – Stand out of the "Usual"

5. Dig up the true meaning of "Dieting"

In a past survey, it was reported that almost 60% of Americans are either obese or gaining weight at a high rate. The Same survey reported that out of all dieting attempts, 90% end up to be a failure. These figures are of a society where there is a whole industry pertain to dieting products and exercise aids.

The word "dieting" is quite familiar to all of us, especially women. Women usually have a history of pursuing variable and trendiest "diets." They start it with a passion and motivation, follow the diet and shed off some initial pounds. With the passage of time, the downfall starts and motivation for dieting starts fading off. Women usually regain the lost weight at this stage and some may even gain more than the previous number of pounds. So the question arises about the ineffectiveness of these diets. But in reality, it is more of a psychological game.

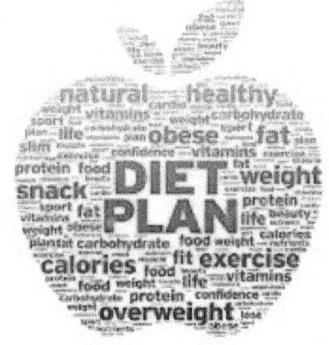

If we relate the dieting perspective with the psychological issues of a person and especially of a woman, we will see following chief issues.

➤ **Unrealistic Expectations**

Apart from the inner mental model, it is somewhat related to untrue marketing campaigns, the diets usually claim unrealistic results and women buy and follow he diets with the expectation that the same results will be achieved. For example, the diet packages may claim that lose 10 pounds within 5 days and a woman starts believing that after these 5 days her life will be at ease.

➤ Rigid Rules

When a diet plan is too rigid to follow, it is hard to continue it with full motivation. Especially if a person had been into excessive eating, he or she will need extra will power to continue these diets with rigid rules.

➤ Elimination of specific nutrients

The market is full of fat-free, carbohydrate free or protein-free diets, so subtracting whole nutrient out of your life is really had to pursue.

➤ Defining a Beginning and an End

Women usually pursue dieting with some definite view. The common examples are, "I am going for a diet from this Monday." Dieting cannot be pursued with these definite markings.

6. Understand the barriers to "thinness"

In this society, everyone wants to be the first one in the list. This over emphasis on the attainment of best possible has made us look for ultimate ideals. Same is the case with the ability to look good. We have started focusing on outlook so much that it has led to a never-ending struggle of looking good.

➢ The need to Redefine thinness:

There is a difference between being healthy and being lean. If you are underweight, look slim but your internal body systems are weak, it will surely lead towards a number of body issues. The top results will be a loss of immunity which can drag to a number of dangerous results. So there is a need to define and prioritize thinness.

➢ Inability to see accurate self-image:

Women are sometimes unable to self the accurate self-image. It is because of their insecurities and lack of confidence. Sometimes women are having a group of friends having an extra slim figure. This put them in a situation which blurs their accurate image. They cannot see their inner beauty and outer magnificence and tart struggling for the same figure; an accurate self-image can keep you away from the unneeded struggles.

➢ Formulate a personal solution for thinness:

When the above two steps of defining the thinness with reference to an accurate self-image will be completed, you can get into the step of forming a customized solution for weight loss. It will help you to stay away from the rule of thumb type diets and exercise plans. Most of the weight loss activities result in faded results because they have been designed with a general perception about obesity and weight gain. Customized solutions always yield better results.

7. Psychological deprivation cycle

It is an important psychological hack which can make you understand the real cause of your failure for not being able to get desired results.

➢ Rules:

The first thing which is followed din case of diet or exercise is to set up "rules". These are like the judgmental phrases, depicting the goodness or badness of a particular behavior.

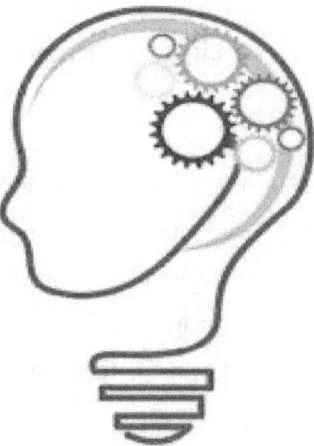

➢ Breaking the rules

Under the effect of these rules, the person will see certain food as either good or bad. For example under your diet rule brownies were bad for weight loss. Now you were on a get together hand your find has served you the brownies. What will you do? Most probably you will eat. It is also because you were a lover of brownies.

➤ Psychological deprivation:

Although you will eat brownies but your mind will keep on signaling that you have broken the rule. It will send disappointment signals to the brain and you will feel low about your weight loss struggle. Eventually, there will be no motivation left.

It is better to cherish your mind with loss connections rather than getting into hard and fast rules.

Chapter 4 – Nothing Stands Impossible

8. Always remember about inaccurate comparisons

One of the biggest mistakes which lead women to suffer from unsuccessful weight loss venture is the tendency to indulge in inaccurate comparisons, under the influence of these incorrect comparisons women tend to feel discontented and discouraged.

➢ Illusions about ideals

We being suspected to illusions, sometimes see the outer shell of any entity. Women see models, actors, and fellows who have unusually slim bodies. But we never know, from what they are 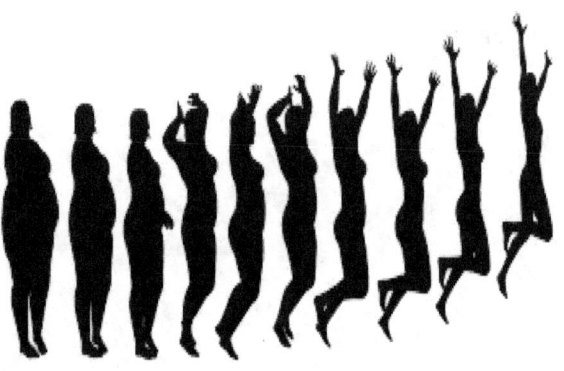 suffering from. Unusual leanness may be the result of some hidden disease or it may have been a gift of genes. So women just start the struggle for reaching the ideals with a false illusion of their perfection. Get rid of this false illusion about ideals or you may render never ending disappointment

➤ Refigure the ideal

As far as weight loss is concerned, women are mostly concerned with weight loss because of their possessiveness to beauty, outlook and a slim figure. However, it is just an incomplete view. A healthier and accurately working body is much more needed. If you weigh lesser than your age, it can be a signal of some hidden disease. In order to achieve successful weight loss, it is necessary to compare your performance with the most optimum solution which can have long-lasting benefits for you.

➤ Everyone is "one" in a million

One of the biggest issues in weight loss of women is their relative approach, they need to understand their uniqueness and their individuality, without which success is not possible, and this uniqueness needs to be considered at every step, from crafting diet plan to making an exercise routine. Even the ideal weight cannot be same for two persons. So sometimes which a woman is labeling as unsuccessful weight loss may be a successful one, under the specific contextual and surrounding factors.

9. Focus on self-monitoring

This is the biggest hack which can reveal miracles. No one can make you follow the path of weight loss, except yourself. Under the influence of self-monitoring you can achieve a number of useful benefits.

- ➤ If you had been into compulsive or Binging or eating, only self-monitoring can stop you. Eventually, the results start to appear as more obvious and clear. Compulsive eating is usually done without restriction so the self-restriction can act as a moderator for this relationship.

- ➤ Self-monitoring will also keep you away from Overeating till it diminishes away fully.

- ➤ Under the self-monitoring effect, the psychological deprivation cycle will get slower as you will not feel an external check on your activities. There will be a "no rule" policy" which will make you feel more satisfied with the results.

- ➤ Under self-monitoring excessive eating will get diminished and eventually the extra pounds will be lost sooner. Sam will be the case of going to exercise or gym.

- ➤ When ideal weight will be achieved self-monitoring can help you to maintain this weight throughout because maintenance is also a motivational task.

10. Build Strongest support system

Throughout this book, we have mentioned that losing weight is surely challenging. It is quite a long way to go. Throughout this venture, there come unlimited challenges and hardships which make a person to go on the back foot. All psychological aspects discussed above were related to individual personality but this last hack is from a social perspective. We all need t support each other for making up healthier society

➢ Generate positive energy

Try to get in touch with the strongest support system, the members of this support system can be your friends or your colleagues or your family members. But the eventual purpose of this support system is to make you continue your struggles. This support system extends positive energy which is needed during weight loss. Weight loss is usually accompanied by lack of confidence and determination but positive energy can enhance the strength.

➢ Constant motivation

When constant energy is dissipated, the eventual result is motivation. women usually lack the motivation, although they may be following the ideal diet plans and exercise routine but with a lack of motivation, they feel disappointed and unsuccessful. Under the effect of motivation, any weight loss venture can turn out to be a real miracle.

Conclusion

The human mind is unveiling the hidden realities confined within the internal and external systems of human body. The research and intellectual efforts of the human race have uncovered a lot of hidden realities present in the surrounding. Same is the case of knowing details about the internal system of human body and mind. The overall healthy human body is governed by a number of connected and intermingled factors, which pertain to both physical and psychological factors. It is because of this deeper knowledge that we are better able to address the issues of modern-day human beings. Deeper understanding has led us to entertain the unattended corners of human life.

When it comes to overall body wellness and outlook, one of the most reported issues for modern-day population is the increasingly high rate of obesity. Almost all sorts of efforts are put forward to overcome obesity but it has entered after a change in the overall eating habits as well as in the living standards of modern men. So fighting for it is not easy. Many people have reported that despite continuous efforts in the form of diet plans and excessive workout, the results have been disappointing. Among these people, a greater segment comprises of women population. After researching on this disappointment scientists have come to the point that psychological factors are also involved in weight loss issues. This book is written to cater the psychological domain of weight loss. The particular audience of this book is the female segment of the population, who is usually more concerned towards weight loss issues.

FREE Bonus Reminder

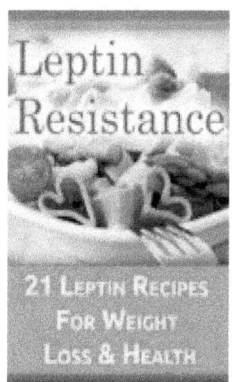

If you have not grabbed it yet, please go ahead and download your special bonus report *"Leptin Resistance. 21 Leptin Recipes For Weight Loss & Healthy Living"*.

Simply Click the Button Below

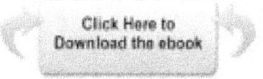

OR **Go to This Page**

http://easyweightlossway.com/free/

BONUS #2: More Free & Discounted Books

Do you want to receive more Free & Discounted Books?

We have a mailing list where we send out our new Books when they go free or with a discount on Kindle. Click on the link below to sign up for Free & Discount Book Promotions.

=> Sign Up for Free & Discount Book Promotions <=

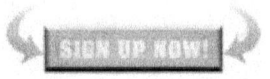

OR Go to this URL

http://zbit.ly/1WBb1Ek

www.ingramcontent.com/pod-product-compliance
Lightning Source LLC
Chambersburg PA
CBHW072023290526
45787CB00014B/1765